EXERCISES FOR
FIBROMYALGIA

William Smith

with Contributions by Jo Brielyn

Foreword by Zinovy Meyler, D.O.

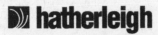

hatherleigh

))) hatherleigh

Hatherleigh Press is committed to preserving and protecting the natural resources of the earth. Environmentally responsible and sustainable practices are embraced within the company's mission statement.

Visit us at www.hatherleighpress.com and register online for free offers, discounts, special events, and more.

Library of Congress Cataloging-in-Publication Data is available.
ISBN: 978-1-57826-361-5

Cover Design by Heather Daugherty
Interior Design by Nick Macagnone
Photography by Catarina Astrom

Printed in the United States

10 9 8 7 6 5 4 3 2

Disclaimer
Consult your physician before beginning any exercise program. The author and publisher of this book and workout disclaim any liability, personal or professional, resulting from the misapplication of any of the following procedures described in this publication.

www.hatherleighpress.com

Table of Contents

FOREWORD

It hasn't been that long since the diagnosis of fibromyalgia was similar to saying to a patient, "I don't know what is wrong with you, but you're in pain." Fibromyalgia has been studied for a long time and descriptions of the syndrome appear in medical literature as early as the 1800s. Throughout history, there are accounts of people with symptoms that are strikingly similar to what we diagnose today as fibromyalgia. Some historians believe that early accounts of symptoms of widespread pain and sleep disturbances can be found in the Old Testament. For several centuries, widespread pain was called rheumatism, then muscular rheumatism. In the early 1900s, the term fibrositis replaced previous names and only in 1976 did we start using the term fibromyalgia to denote the many facets of this syndrome. It was not until the 1980s that we began to find evidence that there is a connection between fibromyalgia and other similar conditions.

In 2007, the first FDA-approved medication for the treatment of fibromyalgia became available. Since then, the research has been ongoing and shows significant promise for practitioners (like myself) and, more importantly, for patients whose lives have been altered by the syndrome. As our understanding grows, there is also some growth of controversy regarding the methods of treatment as well as those applied to the research itself. However, one approach has been able to stand the test of time and science, and that approach is exercise. Of course, people with fibromyalgia face unique challenges when it comes to exercise. Whereas some people can "grin and bear it" and "exercise through the pain," people with fibromyalgia know all too well that you can't simply work through it, or you will often pay the price with a flare of pain later.

Studies consistently show that exercise helps restore the body's neurochemical balance, boost energy, restore sleep, and overall improve the emotional state. As medical practitioners, we see both great results with exercise and, at times, aversion to it due to a negative prior experience and exacerbation of symptoms. It is this double-edged sword that patients and we as physicians face in using therapeutic exercise in the treatment of fibromyalgia. On the one hand, exercise is another form of exertion for someone who already has decreased endurance, fatigue, and disturbed sleep. For someone with fibromyalgia, to take on an exercise routine means overcoming the above barriers, only to face the next question: How do I exercise so that I get the benefits without getting the unwanted increase in fatigue and pain? What are the appropriate exercises and where do I start?

In *Exercise for Fibromyalgia,* prominent trainer, author, and rehabilitative specialist William Smith has put forth a book that details the theory of exercise in the context of the treatment of fibromyalgia. Medicine as a whole is beginning to combine clinical experience with empirical evidence, showing the science behind the wonder of appropriate therapeutic exercise. Will's efforts in combining clinical experience and scientific knowledge provide a practical application of exercise in treatment of this syndrome. It is a much-needed roadmap in the maze that can be fibromyalgia.

The book you are holding in your hands will prove an invaluable resource for the community that encompasses people diagnosed with fibromyalgia and for medical practitioners undertaking the treatment of people suffering from its multitude of symptoms. We are seeing more and more that this multifaceted syndrome requires an approach that is most in line with the physiology and biochemistry of our bodies. Appropriate exercise is the most efficient way to address this. This book will help you develop the exercise routine right for you and get you on your way to less pain and more gain!

—Zinovy Meyler, D.O

Co-Director, Interventional Spine Program
Princeton Spine and Joint Center

INTRODUCTION

If you are dealing with the fatigue, muscle pain, and tender points often associated with fibromyalgia, exercise may seem like the last thing you want to consider doing. You may be surprised to learn, however, that getting active and adopting a regular exercise regimen is exactly what you need. Instead of increasing your aches and pains, the proper types of exercise will actually make you feel better while helping to fight off many of your fibromyalgia symptoms and flares. The value of physical activity for the management of fibromyalgia, coupled with a healthy diet and lifestyle, is the focus of this book.

New findings suggest that physical activity such as stretching, strength training, and walking are beneficial in improving the physical, social, and emotional functioning of fibromyalgia patients. Other studies show that low-impact aerobic exercises—such as Pilates, yoga, tai chi, and water therapy—are also effective in building and strengthening muscles and reducing the symptoms associated with fibromyalgia.

To achieve maximum benefits, focus on including these three main types of exercises in your exercise program:

Strengthening exercises: Strengthening exercises are intended to build the strong tendons and muscles necessary to support the joints. Of course, it is important that you use caution when performing strength-building exercises to avoid causing injury or inflicting further pain on your body.

Conditioning exercises: Exercises like walking, biking, and swimming are good examples of conditioning exercises. They strengthen and tone your muscles while also increasing your endurance and coordination. Conditioning exercises are also helpful if you are trying to lose weight.

Stretching (or range of motion) exercises: Exercises in this category involve moving joints through their full range of motion, or as far as possible without pain. They help promote flexibility in the muscles and loosen stiffness often connected with fibromyalgia.

CHAPTER ONE

What is Fibromyalgia?

Fibromyalgia is a complex chronic pain disorder that can cause great physical and mental distress. People with fibromyalgia generally endure long-term fatigue and musculoskeletal pain in joints, tendons, muscles, and other soft tissues throughout their entire body. The sometimes debilitating syndrome gets its name from "fibro" which means fibrous tissue (like ligaments and tendons), "my" meaning muscles, and "algia" which means pain.

The National Institute of Arthritis and Musculoskeletal and Skin Diseases (NIAMS) reported that fibromyalgia affects approximately 5 million people 18 years of age or older in the United States alone. Yet fibromyalgia (which is also sometimes referred to as fibromyalgia syndrome, fibrositis, or fibromyositis) is classified as a *syndrome,* not a disease. To be considered a disease, there must be a definite cause, or causes, as well as signs and symptoms that are clearly identified. Unfortunately, that is not the case with fibromyalgia. Because of this, the syndrome has been dubbed the "Great Imitator."

1

While widespread pain is universal to all people who live with fibromyalgia, the symptoms and severity of them are varied. Even when two people experience the same symptoms, they tend to manifest themselves differently in each person. Also, fibromyalgia patients experience numerous symptoms and medical issues that frequently occur together but do not have one specific cause that can be pinpointed. Many of the symptoms overlap with ones present in other conditions, which can lead to extensive and costly medical exploration and frustration for patients. For these reasons, it takes an average of five years for a person to get a correct diagnosis of fibromyalgia.

Common Symptoms of Fibromyalgia

Chronic widespread pain in the body: Pain that travels to all four quadrants of the body and persists for three or more months is the primary symptom found in people with fibromyalgia. The pain varies from sharp shooting pains to deep aches and twitches in the muscles.

Pain or tenderness in the main tender points of the body when pressure is applied to them: Tender points are located in the soft tissue on the back of the neck, shoulders, chest, elbows, hips, buttocks, lower back, shins, and knees. The pain originates from those points and then spreads out. To receive a diagnosis of fibromyalgia, an individual must experience tenderness or pain in at least 11 of the 18 tender points.

Moderate to extreme fatigue and poor stamina that may interfere with daily activities: Fatigue is a major complaint among individuals with fibromyalgia. It is often compared to how one would feel after working long hours, battling the flu, or losing a lot of sleep. Fatigue associated with fibromyalgia is a tiredness that lingers even when the person is rested.

Sleep problems: Many people with fibromyalgia have trouble falling asleep and staying asleep for a long length of time. They often complain of still feeling tired when they wake up.

Stiffness in the morning: More than 75 percent of people with fibromyalgia experience some level of stiffness in the muscles and joints of the back, arms, and legs after first getting up in the morning. It may last for a few minutes, several hours, or in severe cases, persist for the majority of the day.

Tingling, numbness, or burning sensation in the body, especially the hands and feet: These sensations, called *paresthesia*, occur at irregular times. Paresthesia may last for a few minutes or can be constant.

Sensitivity to environmental sensations like touch, sound, and light: Bright lights, loud noises, and sometimes physical touch can trigger pain and cognitive difficulties for fibromyalgia sufferers. Sensory sensitivity varies from day to day.

"Fibro fog" or "brain fog": Fibromyalgia sufferers often deal with cognitive difficulties such as impaired concentration and memory. This is sometimes referred to as being in a "fibro fog."

Dizziness: Over two-thirds of people with fibromyalgia report regular bouts of lightheadedness or unsteadiness. Dizziness can also lead to fainting spells and falls, so it is important to exercise caution to avoid injuries.

Migraines and other types of chronic headaches: Statistics show that about 75 percent of people with fibromyalgia suffer from chronic headaches. Migraines, tension headaches, and combination headaches—a combination of migraine and tension headaches—are linked to fibromyalgia.

Dysmenorrhea: Since people with fibromyalgia have a higher sensitivity to pain, female patients often experience dysmenorrhea as a symptom. Dysmenorrhea is a disorder that causes extreme pain in the abdomen, pelvis, and other areas of the body during the menstrual cycle.

Problems with coordination: People with fibromyalgia often experience problems with coordination and balance, which increases the risks of falling.

Palpitations: Palpitations are another common symptom found in fibromyalgia patients. They are sensations that the heart is racing and are felt in the chest, throat, or neck.

Jaw pain: At least one-quarter of people with fibromyalgia deal with pain in the jaw and face, a symptom that is called *temporomandibular joint dysfunction*. The pain is generally related to the muscles and ligaments surrounding the jaw joint, not the actual joint.

Common Conditions That Overlap with Fibromyalgia

Many individuals who are diagnosed with fibromyalgia also suffer from other conditions and diseases that may exhibit some of the same symptoms that are associated with fibromyalgia. The ones listed below are some of the most common conditions that overlap with fibromyalgia.

- Lupus
- Arthritis
- Lyme disease
- Irritable bowel syndrome (IBS)
- Irritable bladder
- Temporomandibular joint disorder (TMJ)
- Anxiety
- Chronic back or neck pain
- Chronic fatigue syndrome (CFS)
- Hypothyroidism
- Sleep disorders
- Depression
- Restless Legs Syndrome
- Raynaud's Syndrome

Risk Factors for Fibromyalgia

Although the specific cause of fibromyalgia is still unknown, there are some risk factors that scientists and physicians have been able to link to the syndrome.

Genetics: Studies suggest that there is a genetic component to fibromyalgia. The syndrome is often seen among mothers and their children, in siblings, or among other close family members.

Gender: While the risk of developing fibromyalgia is not exclusive to one gender, there are far more diagnoses reported for women than for men. Approximately 80 percent of patients being treated for fibromyalgia are female. It is not known why this disorder affects women so much more than men.

4

Age: The majority of individuals who are diagnosed with the syndrome are women in their childbearing years, generally between the ages of 20 and 50 years old. Diagnoses do occur among men of those same ages and elderly people, but not nearly as often. While it is not impossible for children to have fibromyalgia, it is rare.

Injury or trauma that affects the central nervous system: Data shows that fibromyalgia often occurs after the individual experiences a physical trauma, like a car accident, surgery, or acute illness. It is believed that injury or trauma that somehow affects the central nervous system may act as a catalyst in the development of the syndrome.

Sleep disorders: Scientists speculate that sleep disorders may be one of the underlying causes of fibromyalgia. A great number of people with fibromyalgia do suffer from sleep disorders and, consequently, become extremely fatigued. Individuals who have been diagnosed with a sleep disorder, such as sleep apnea or insomnia, may be at a higher risk for developing fibromyalgia.

Lupus: Individuals who have been diagnosed with lupus are at increased risk of developing fibromyalgia. Much like fibromyalgia, lupus is a disorder that mainly affects women and produces symptoms of pain and fatigue. Statistics prove that around 30 percent of people who have lupus are later diagnosed with fibromyalgia.

Osteoarthritis: It is still unclear why, but there also seems to be a link between people diagnosed with osteoarthritis and fibromyalgia. Osteoarthritis, a variety of arthritis that causes degeneration of the joints, causes pain and disability to sufferers. If you have osteoarthritis, your risk for developing fibromyalgia is higher. About 10 to 15 percent of osteoarthritis patients also have fibromyalgia.

Ankylosing Spondylitis: Ankylosing spondylitis is another type of arthritis that puts its sufferers at a higher risk for fibromyalgia. The condition causes severe back pain and inflammation in the joints between the pelvis and spine.

Viral or bacterial infection: Fibromyalgia also seems to be triggered by both bacterial and viral infections.

Aggravating Factors that Affect Fibromyalgia Pain

Fibromyalgia symptoms tend to occur in cycles. You may find that your fibromyalgia symptoms are fine one day and then increase dramatically the next. This is called a *fibromyalgia flare.* There are some environmental, physical, and emotional factors that may trigger a flare and increase the pain associated with fibromyalgia. In time, you will start to recognize the factors that are catalysts for your flares. By learning how to regulate or make accommodations for these factors, you may be able to keep your pain levels lower and reduce the frequency and severity of your fibromyalgia flares.

Below are some common factors which are known to aggravate fibromyalgia symptoms:

- Cold or damp weather
- Humidity
- Alcohol
- Physical fatigue
- Mental fatigue
- Anxiety
- Stress
- Too much physical activity or overexertion
- Physical inactivity
- Lack of restorative sleep
- Insomnia

You can contact these organizations to learn more about fibromyalgia, ask specific questions, or receive additional information:

Fibromyalgia.com
Website: www.fibromyalgia.com

Fibromyalgia Network
Toll-free phone number: (800) 853-2929
Website: www.fmnetnews.com

Fibromyalgia Symptoms
Website: www.fibromyalgia-symptoms.org

National Fibromyalgia Association (NFA)
Phone number: (714) 921-0150
Website: www.fmaware.org

The National Institute of Arthritis and Musculoskeletal and Skin Diseases (NIAMS)
Toll-free phone number: (877) 22-NIAMS or (877) 226-4267
Website: www.niams.nih.gov

U.S. National Library of Medicine
Website: www.ncbi.nlm.nih.gov/pubmedhealth

CHAPTER TWO

What the New Studies Say

While scientists have not yet found a cure for fibromyalgia and much of the syndrome remains a mystery for the time being, more effective ways to diagnose and treat the syndrome are being created. Research efforts for fibromyalgia are expanding. There are currently over 4,000 studies and reports related to fibromyalgia that have been published, in comparison with the meager 200 that were available back in 1990. Without a cure, treatment options for fibromyalgia must focus primarily on relieving the symptoms and improving the daily functioning of patients.

Despite the steps forward that have been made in the last twenty years, fibromyalgia remains a challenge. Clinical studies have revealed that the greatest improvements are made for fibromyalgia patients when they are involved with a balanced treatment plan. A varied treatment that combines medications, alternative therapies, and lifestyle changes like nutrition and exercise can drastically reduce the individual's fibromyalgia symptoms and improve the quality of life.

One such study was conducted by a team of Boston researchers from Beth Israel Deaconess Medical Center, Brigham and Women's Hospital, and Harvard Medical School. Daniel S. Rooks, ScD and his team set out to evaluate and compare four common self-management interventions for fibromyalgia patients. Of the 207 women they recruited for the study, 135 of them completed the 16-week intervention period and participated in a follow-up assessment. The team determined that the group that participated in a strength training/aerobics/flexibility exercise class and the Arthritis Foundation Fibromyalgia Self-Help Course (FSHC) achieved the most improvement in key symptoms and physical, emotional, and social functions. When the report was published in the *Archives of Internal Medicine*, the conclusion was that the "… study suggests that progressive walking, simple strength training movements, and stretching activities are effective at improving physical, emotional and social function, key symptoms, and self-efficacy in women with fibromyalgia who are being actively treated with medication. Furthermore, the benefits of exercise are enhanced when combined with targeted self-management education."

New Medications for Fibromyalgia Relief

Medications to improve sleep and control pain are often prescribed for people with fibromyalgia. Pain relievers, muscle relaxants, anti-seizure drugs, sleeping aids, and antidepressants are often used to relieve symptoms of the syndrome. Since June of 2007, three new medications to aid in fibromyalgia treatment have been approved by the U.S. Food and Drug Administration: Lyrica (pregabalin), Cymbalta (duloxetine HC1), and Savella (milnacipran HC1). Other medications for fibromyalgia sufferers are also currently in development.

Use of Natural and Alternative Therapies

Many individuals with fibromyalgia also find relief from symptoms with the help of natural and alternative methods of therapy. These types of treatments can be used on their own or in combination with traditional therapies. It is advisable, however, to consult with your doctor to make sure that your choice of method, such as medicinal herbs, will not negatively interact with your prescription medicines.

Did you know?

- Fibromyalgia researchers and specialists estimate that the healthcare costs associated with fibromyalgia in the United States are between $12 and $14 billion each year.

- It takes an individual an average of 5 years to get a true diagnosis of fibromyalgia.

- Fibromyalgia accounts for 1 to 2 percent of America's overall productivity loss.

- Studies show that, at any given time, approximately 25 percent of fibromyalgia patients receive some form of disability compensation.

- The National Fibromyalgia Association reports that about 5 to 7 percent of Americans are affected by fibromyalgia.

- Data indicates that African-American women are more likely to suffer from fibromyalgia than their Caucasian counterparts.

- Almost 90 percent of people who have fibromyalgia also suffer from a sleep disorder, severe fatigue, or both.

Below are some natural and alternative therapies commonly used by fibromyalgia patients:
- Massage
- Acupuncture
- Acupressure
- Myofascial release
- Chiropractic treatments
- Herbal supplements
- Yoga and meditation
- Light therapy
- Osteopathy
- Support groups

Creating a personalized treatment plan that includes the proper blend of medical and/or natural and alternative therapies, a well-balanced diet, good sleep habits, and a smart exercise routine will help reduce and manage the pain and symptoms of your fibromyalgia to help improve your quality of life.

CHAPTER THREE

The Key to Long-Term Health

Pharmaceuticals and therapies for treating fibromyalgia are improving continually, but they alone are not enough. Lifestyle factors like proper nutrition, healthy sleep habits, a nd regular exercise are a vital part of dealing with your fibromyalgia in a proactive manner.

Sleep

Sleep is becoming an endangered resource. We live busier and busier lives that motivate us to work harder and longer. Sleep deprivation has been linked to increased risk of fibromyalgia, slower reflexes, negative mental functioning in the brain, and elevated stress levels. Sleep apnea, a severe sleep disorder that causes people to stop breathing (for up to 10 seconds) while they are asleep, is a major risk factor for fibromyalgia. Other sleep problems often found among people with fibromyalgia include insomnia, difficulty falling asleep, frequently awakening in the night, and restless leg syndrome.

The National Institutes of Health estimate that 60 million Americans have insomnia frequently or for extended periods of time. The NIH indicates sleep problems affect virtually every aspect of day-to-day living including mood, mental alertness, work performance, and energy level.

Sleep deprivation has direct links to impairments in concentration, memory, and cognitive function. Sleep acts as medicine for the brain, healing brain tissue that is under constant stress, both good and bad. Think of the brain as a computer that must shut down and "re-boot." This allows for the downtime the body needs for rest, recovery, and stimulating the five stages of sleeping cycles culminating in Rapid Eye Movement (REM) and Non Rapid Eye Movement (NREM) sleep. Inadequate sleep also acts as a trigger for many fibromyalgia symptoms. Improving your sleep can help decrease the frequency and intensity of "fibro fog," fatigue, pain, and anxiety/depression related to your fibromyalgia.

Research recommends we get between 7–8 hours of sleep every night. Is this realistic? We know that sleep and memory are intimately linked, but what if someone is not getting their daily dose? Drugs, herbal remedies, and sleep clinics are often recommended.

Simple steps to promote quality sleep include the following:
- Avoid stimulants such as caffeine, alcohol, and chocolates before bed.
- Schedule the most vigorous workouts earlier in the day.
- Try to go to bed every night at the same time, take naps at regular intervals, and avoid sleeping during the day if you truly are not tired.

Stress Relievers: Breathing, Meditation, and Visual Imagery

The manner in which you respond to stress may increase your risk of developing fibromyalgia, exacerbate existing symptoms, or induce a fibromyalgia flare. For instance, stress often prompts more instances of sleep problems, overeating, abuse of alcohol and illicit drugs, and smoking.

A Breathing Exercise: The Gateway to Daily Meditation

Focusing on the breath is one of the most common and fundamental techniques for accessing the meditative state. Breath is a deep rhythm of the body that connects us intimately with the world around us. Learn these steps, and then practice them as a regular breathing exercise.

Close your eyes, breathe deeply and regularly, and observe your breath as it flows in through the nose and out through the mouth. Give your full attention to the breath as it comes in and goes out. Store your breath in the belly, not the chest, between inhales and exhales. Whenever you find your attention wandering away from your breath, gently pull it back to the rising and falling of the breath via the belly.

Inhale through your nose slowly and deeply, feeling the lower chest and abdomen inflate like a balloon. Hold for five seconds. Exhale deeply, deflating the lower chest and abdomen like an emptying balloon. Hold for five seconds. Do this five times, and then allow your breathing to return to a normal rhythm.

You will begin to feel a change come over your entire body. Gradually you will become less aware of your breathing, but not captured in your stream of consciousness. Consciousness is encouraged on the whole, but we often are too alert and hyper-stimulated via TV, caffeine, and family life, just to name a few. By performing deep breathing for five minutes daily, you will become more centered inward. You will just live "in the moment," in your own skin.

Benefits of a simple breathing exercise throughout the day include:
- Calming
- "Re-centering" one's thoughts
- Increase in oxygenated blood flow and improved efficiency in expiring carbon dioxide
- Decreased levels of fatigue later in the day, reducing any "heavy" feeling in the legs
- Reduction in stress, anxiety, and depression
- Aiding in pain management and decreasing fibromyalgia symptoms
- Reduced severity, duration, and incidences of migraines and other chronic headaches

Increasing oxygenated blood via deep breathing can decrease muscle pains, especially in the postural muscles (back and neck muscles), and can help counteract chronic stressors such as sitting or standing in static positions for extended periods of time.

Deep Breathing
Practice deep breathing as a form of relaxation before bed. Slow, deep breathing is an excellent way to slow the heart rate and contemplate the day's events. Focus on breathing in through the nose and out through the mouth.

Simple Stress Reliever

Looking for a simple, healthy way to help get through the day? Try breathing exercises—a wonderfully effective way to reduce stress, maintain focus, and feel energized. Exhaling completely is one breathing exercise to try. It can promote deeper breathing and better health.

Give it a try: Simply take a deep breath, let it out effortlessly, and then squeeze out a little more. Doing this regularly will help build up the muscles between your ribs, and your exhalations will soon become deeper and longer. Start by practicing this exhalation exercise consciously, and before long it will become a healthy, unconscious habit.

Hydration: Water Intake and Fibromyalgia

Hydrate, Hydrate, Hydrate! 60 percent of your body is water. That means you should take in half your body weight, or 25–30 percent, through your diet. This is equivalent to six to eight 8–ounce glasses of water per day. Ask yourself, do you do this? Keeping bottled water on hand when traveling or during physical activity will increase the likeliness of fluid intake.

Oddly enough, you should drink when you're not thirsty. This is because, by the time you experience thirst, your body has already been deprived of the hydration it needs for some time. Remember, don't wait until you're parched to drink water; rather, be sure to drink water before that occurs.

In addition, start to keep tabs on visible feedback including urine color, skin pliability, and normal sweating. Urine color should be pale to light in color. Skin pliability should stretch and return to normal texture immediately. Sweating can be an additional indication of proper hydration. Sweating during exercise and physical activity is normal and expected. Exercise without sweating, while it does happen, is not a regular occurrence.

The Dangers of Dehydration

Difficulty concentrating, fatigue, and stiffness in body tissues may be caused by dehydration. The general recommendation is six to eight glasses of water per day, yet with elderly populations this amount is easily decreased by one to two glasses. Low hydration is a concern even in inactive populations that do not physically exert themselves beyond activities of daily living. Basic physiological functions including digestion, perspiration, urination, and renal function all require fluids.

> Water intake is important to improving your life with fibromyalgia. When your body doesn't get enough water, your brain becomes less active, concentration is impaired, and your body feels fatigued—all issues that people with fibromyalgia are already more prone to experiencing. Proper hydration reduces these complications and also helps keep your immune system at its prime, which in turn puts less stress on your body and eases many of the symptoms associated with the disease.

Making Smart Food Choices

A healthy, balanced diet is an essential element of the treatment plan for fibromyalgia. A diet that is plentiful in foods like fruits and vegetables will supply your body with antioxidants, fiber, and many other nutrients and vitamins it needs. It is also important to be aware of foods that serve as triggers for your fibromyalgia flares and adjust your diet to eliminate or reduce them. Keeping a food diary is an effective way to help you identify your pain triggers and which foods make you feel good.

Common Food Triggers for Fibromyalgia

- Caffeine
- Artificial sweeteners like aspartame
- Soy
- Yogurt
- Aged or blue cheeses
- Yellow cheeses
- Red wine
- Beer
- Chocolate
- Processed meats
- Yeast
- Snack foods like chips and pretzels
- Chinese food (or any other food with MSG)

The following are some natural ways to add important vitamins and nutrients to your diet, which can help boost and maintain your health.

Natural Sources of Calcium:
- Milk
- Sardines
- Salmon
- Any seafood that contains bones
- Turnip greens
- Spinach
- Kale
- Broccoli
- Nuts (almonds, Brazil nuts, and pecans)
- Legumes (peas, lentils, and beans)

Natural Sources of Vitamin D:
- Sunlight
- Eggs
- Milk
- Tuna
- Liver oils
- Mackerel
- Cod
- Sea bass

Natural Sources of Vitamin A:
- Milk
- Eggs
- Yellow vegetables (summer squash)
- Carrots
- Liver
- Green leafy vegetables (kale, spinach, greens, and romaine lettuce)
- Fruits (cantaloupe, tomatoes, and apricots)

Natural Sources of Vitamin B12:
- Liver
- Lean beef
- Clams
- Salmon
- Haddock
- Trout
- Cheese
- Eggs

Natural Sources of Vitamin C:
- Citrus
- Papayas
- Green vegetables
- Berries

Natural Sources of Vitamin E:
- Dark green leafy vegetables
- Nuts
- Vegetable oils
- Whole grains
- Wheat germ

Natural Sources of Vitamin K:
- Seeds
- Eggs
- Dairy products
- Broccoli
- Brussels sprouts
- Chick peas

Natural Sources of Potassium:
- Milk
- Green leafy vegetables (romaine lettuce, spinach, Swiss chard, and greens)
- Broccoli
- Lentils
- Winter squash
- Fruits (tomatoes, cantaloupe, avocado, oranges, and strawberries)
- Snapper
- Halibut
- Scallops
- Soy
- Potatoes (white and sweet varieties)

Natural Sources of Copper:
- Vegetables
- Liver
- Legumes
- Nuts
- Seeds
- Beans

Natural Sources of Magnesium:
- Brazil nuts
- Seeds (sunflower seeds, pumpkin seeds, and sesame seeds)
- Bananas
- Legumes
- Tofu
- Green leafy vegetables (spinach, Swiss chard, and kelp)
- Whole grains (barley, brown rice, and oats)

Daily Tips to Stay Healthy

1. Stretch for five minutes before getting out of bed in the morning to prepare your muscles for movement.
2. Drink one large glass of water in the morning to stabilize your morning eating habits. By replenishing your body first thing in the morning, your regulatory systems, namely heart rate and blood pressure, will stay increasingly balanced.

3. Eat 300–400 calories for breakfast. Research has shown that eating breakfast improves memory performance.
4. Healthy lunch foods can easily be made to order at local restaurants. Pick steamed and broiled foods over fried. Gastro-Intestinal (GI) irritability (a common symptom associated with fibromyalgia) can be exacerbated by fried and processed foods.
5. Mid-afternoon is a perfect time to have a moderate carbohydrate/moderate protein-based snack or drink. An example would be a smoothie of dark berries (using milk instead of yogurt) with whey protein blended with water.
6. If eating dinner around 5:00 or 6:00, it can be on the heavier side, whereas dinners at 7:00 or later should be on the lighter side. If you know you will be having dinner later in the day, add another serving of milk instead of water to your smoothie, increasing the total caloric intake for your mid-afternoon snack. This will keep you from getting hungry as the day goes on.
7. Take a walk after dinner, but wait 20–30 minutes after eating. Stimulating blood flow through aerobically-based movements that are low-impact (not running) aids in the digestive process. Giving 30 minutes allows the food to settle.
8. Write a short to-do list before going to bed. Keep your list to three priority items if you do not work and 1–2 priority items if you have a full-time occupation.
9. Practice deep breathing as a form of relaxation before bed. Deep breathing is an excellent way to slow the heart rate. Focus on breathing in through the nose and out through the mouth.

Tips for Taking Control of Your Fibromyalgia

Maintain good posture: Fibromyalgia treatments can help people relax their muscles and reduce their pain level, but poor posture practices (such as slouching over a computer, hunching over the steering wheel while driving, and lifting improperly) are lifelong habits that can actually counteract your treatment efforts and cause more pain. Poor posture contributes to muscle pain and stiffness.

Make your breathing count: Take deep breaths that cause your abdomen to expand when you inhale and contract when you exhale. Shallow breaths deprive your body and its muscles of the proper amount of oxygen. Not getting enough oxygen may cause tender points in the body and can also increase the aches and pains associated with fibromyalgia. Insufficient levels of oxygen intensify fatigue, too.

Be prepared for seasonal changes: Since fibromyalgia flares are often exacerbated by rapid changes in temperature, moisture, and barometric pressure, it is wise to be prepared for the seasonal changes. Watch the weather and dress accordingly. For instance, wear layers of clothing and stay away from drafty areas in the cooler months. In the summer months, try to limit your time outside when it is hot and humid. Also, avoid sitting too close to heaters or air conditioners.

Try to limit infections: Individuals with fibromyalgia often seem to be more prone to common colds and viral and bacterial infections. This may be due, in part, to the fact that sleep deprivation has weakened their immune systems. Any new infections add more stress on your immune system and can cause your fibromyalgia symptoms to get worse. This is another reason why practicing good hygiene, maintaining a healthy diet, and promoting a healthy lifestyle are so vital to your well-being.

Make some changes to your lifestyle: There are several facets of your daily life that can affect your fibromyalgia symptoms and may need to be changed. Making these changes can go a long way in improving your health and reducing your pain. Here are a few examples:
- If you smoke, quit. If you don't smoke, then don't start.
- Keep regular hours and try to get the same amount of sleep each night. Avoid staying up too late or getting up too early.
- Eliminate alcoholic beverages, or at least drink them sparingly.
- Work hours that shift from week to week may be difficult for people with fibromyalgia. If your job requires it, try to limit the amount of shift work you do.
- Know your limits. Do not push yourself too hard or overwork your body, physically or mentally.
- Remember to drink adequate amounts of water to stay hydrated, but try to limit how much you drink before bedtime to avoid waking in the night because of a full bladder.

CHAPTER FOUR

Path to Better Health: The Benefits of Exercise

Individuals who deal with the daily muscle aches, fatigue, and other painful symptoms associated with fibromyalgia may cringe at the very thought of increasing exercise and physical activity. It seems to go against logic to exercise more when you are already feeling pain. In fact, before scientific studies and patient success stories proved otherwise, physicians thought the same thing. They also believed that exercise might worsen the disease for their patients. Fibromyalgia patients were told to rest, not to be active.

Yet, the reality is that exercises—the right ones customized to fit individual needs—benefit people with fibromyalgia instead of exacerbating their symptoms.

How Does Exercise Benefit People Living with Fibromyalgia?

Regular exercise boosts the body's endorphins (pain-fighting molecules) and serotonin (the brain chemical that influences moods). An increase in one or both helps to naturally relieve stress, anxiety, and depression which are often

23

symptomatic in individuals with a chronic illness like fibromyalgia. Engaging in exercise improves moods, attitude, and quality of life for individuals.

Other ways exercise benefits people with fibromyalgia:
- Strengthens bones and muscles
- Controls weight and burns calories
- Increases energy levels
- Improves flexibility and range-of-motion in sore joints and muscles
- Increases aerobic ability
- Helps with quality of sleep
- Improves cardiovascular health
- Relieves pain
- Decreases tension and stiffness in muscles

What Kinds of Exercises Are Best for Helping with Fibromyalgia Symptoms?

The exercises found in this book are aimed at increasing flexibility, balance, strength, stability, and mobility for people living with fibromyalgia. Combined with the carefully planned exercise programs and progressions in Chapter 7, the exercises will help reduce symptoms and provide individuals with some control over fibromyalgia pain. Below are a few recommended exercises for each. Please refer to Chapter 6 for a complete list and descriptions of the exercises.

To Improve Mobility:
- Foam Roller Scissor Stretch (page 50)
- Roll and Hold (page 51)
- Ribcage Opener (page 52)
- Prone Extension Lifts (page 54)

To Improve Balance:
- Heel to Toe Rocks (page 55)
- Physio-Ball Walk-Up (page 56)
- Clock Lunge (page 58)
- Doggy Door (page 60)

To Improve Stability:
- Inch Worm Walk-Up (page 61)
- Double Leg Bridge (page 62)
- Pelvic Tilt (page 63)
- Kegel (page 64)

To Improve Flexibility:
- Bent Knee Hamstring (page 65)
- Abductors (page 67)
- Lateral Neck Stretch (page 70)
- Straight Leg Stretch (page 73)

To Improve Strength:
- Lateral Lunge with Shoulder Press (page 74)
- Band Pulls with One Knee Up (page 76)
- Stability Hold in Push-Up (page 80)
- Standard Lunge with Bicep Curl (page 81)

Please remember that practicing moderation and pacing yourself are always important whenever beginning a new exercise routine. Pay attention to your symptoms and take breaks when you need them, but don't give up. The payoff will be more energy, less pain, and a better quality of life.

CHAPTER FIVE

Rules of the Road: Exercise Precautions

In the following chapter, you will find many great exercises that satisfy fibromyalgia patients' need for physical activity, including exercises that improve balance and strength, as well as movement-based exercises. The exercises and Programs found in Chapters 6 and 7 are specially designed to be safe and effective, even for those with recurring pain.

Patients following the Programs in Chapter 7 should not hesitate to tailor the workouts to their own specific needs and abilities by panning through and finding the exercises they really enjoy. These are the exercises you will be more likely to perform with increased regularity and consistency, which are two key factors for achieving a healthier body.

Through performing these exercises, you will be participating in something called *motor learning*. It is important to keep in mind that there will be a learning curve for new physical and mental exercises, which may cause some frustration as you become accustomed to the movements and activities.

The first few weeks of the Program are called the *cognitive (verbal) stage,* during which you will be mentally figuring out what to do. This should last three to four weeks.

During the second learning stage, named the *associative stage,* you should be able to perform the action, but possibly with errors. This should last two to three weeks.

Lastly, the *automatic stage* is when you are able to perform the exercises without error (or, with "great form") and can repeat sets and reps week after week.

Exercise Essentials Checklist

Exercise Preparation

- **Exercise Location:** Is your environment safe, clean, and free of debris?
- **Proper Footwear:** Are you wearing proper athletic footwear?
- **Comfortable Athletic Wear:** Do you have clothes that allow freedom of movement?
- **Hydration:** Be sure to drink six glasses of fluid over the course of your day.

Exercise Equipment

- **Rolled-up towel:** Can be used for resistance training, balancing on the floor, etc.
- **Mirror:** Provides visual feedback on cueing and technique
- **Dumbbells:** 5–10 pound range is generally appropriate
- **Therabands:** Light-colored bands offer less resistance and dark-colored bands offer more resistance
- **Physio-ball:** Inflate the ball to the point where you can press your thumb on the surface without it sinking in
- **Tennis ball or racquet ball:** For hand and foot therapy

Playing it Safe: Important Safety Precautions

Body Positioning: Brace your core, achieve proper alignment, feel the placement of your feet, and always move first from your core before moving your limbs.

Keep a Health Journal: In this journal, you can record how you're feeling on any given day and what activities you did during that time. You should also record what kinds of exercises you did on each day and how you felt during and after your exercise session. Keeping track of this information will help you better understand your own health, which is a crucial step on the road to recovery.

Rate of Perceived Exertion (RPE): You can use the chart below to gauge how hard you are working during your session. The corresponding numerical values may also be helpful for you to record in your Health Journal, if you choose to keep one.

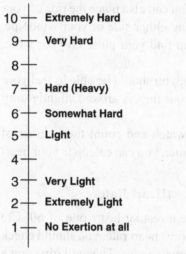

10 — Extremely Hard

9 — Very Hard

8 —

7 — Hard (Heavy)

6 — Somewhat Hard

5 — Light

4 —

3 — Very Light

2 — Extremely Light

1 — No Exertion at all

Talk Test: This is another useful way of determining how hard you are working. As you are exercising, gauge how easily you are able to converse and use the guidelines below to figure out the intensity of your exertion.

If you can carry on a normal conversation while exercising, you are likely working *aerobically,* which means your body is using oxygen as its primary energy source. If you can work aerobically for up to 30-45 minutes, your body will also be using fat as an energy source, which is an excellent foundation for building your exercise program.

Anaerobic work, characterized below as medium intensity, should be introduced eight weeks into your exercise program. Examples include hill walking, bike sprints, etc. When performing anaerobic exercise, you may notice your leg muscles starting to feel a bit tight, your chest will expand, you will begin to sweat, and your heart rate will reach about 40–50 beats above your resting heart rate (see page 30 for more details on determining your heart rate).

Low Intensity: Complete sentences, breathing rate normal
Medium Intensity: Broken sentences, breathing rate slightly labored
High Intensity: Cannot converse, breathing rate labored

Be sure to see your healthcare provider regularly for check-ups.

Determining Your Heart Rate

To determine your heart rate, place the tips of your index and third fingers on your wrist, below the base of your thumb. You can also place the tips of your index and second fingers on your neck, along either side of your windpipe. During exercise, it is recommended that you find your pulse on your wrist, rather than on your neck.

While pressing lightly with your fingers, you should be able to feel your pulse. If you don't feel your pulse, move your fingers around slightly until you find your pulse.

Watch the second hand of a clock or watch and count the number of beats you feel in 10 seconds. Using that number, you can calculate your heart rate with the formula below:

$$\text{(Beats in ten seconds)} \times 6 = \text{(Heart Rate)}$$

Adults over 18 years of age typically have a resting heart rate of 60–100 beats per minute. To better understand your own heart rate, you should check your pulse before, and immediately after, you exercise. This will give you a better idea of what your body normally does at rest, and to what level your heart should be working during an exercise session.

Important Assessments

Medical Tests

Medical tests include blood panels, neurological/reflexive tests, updated family history, stress test, etc. These are tests that your medical provider can provide based upon your clinical assessment of health and risk profile. Maintain an open dialogue your medical practitioner, particularly if you have a history of heart problems.

Fitness Tests (Functional and Physical Assessments)

- **Functional Assessment:** The Functional Assessment will provide you with a direct measurement of how you can improve in your activities of daily living. This includes walking stairs, getting in and out of chairs, etc. Refer to Chapter 7, page 88 for the Functional Assessment.

Calculating Target Heart Rate

Your target heart rate is the level of exertion you should aim for when exercising in order to gain the most benefits from your workout. Your target heart rate is also a useful range for how your body is responding to your workout.

Target heart rate is 60– 80% of your maximum heart rate, depending on what level of exertion you wish to work at.

Different Training Zones
Below is a list of the different levels of exertion and the corresponding percentage you would use to target heart rate:

Recovery Zone - 60% to 70%
Active recovery training should fall into this zone (ideally at the lower end). It's also useful for very early pre-season and closed season cross training when the body needs to recover and replenish.

Aerobic Zone - 70% to 80%
Exercising in this zone will help to develop your aerobic system and, in particular, your ability to transport and utilize oxygen. Continuous or rhythmic endurance training, like running and hiking, should fall under this heart rate zone.

Anaerobic Zone – 80% to 90%
Training in this zone will help to improve your body's ability to deal with lactic acid. It may also help to increase your lactate threshold.

To determine your target heart rate, you can use the formulas below to calculate your maximum heart rate, and to then find your target heart rate.

220 – age = maximum heart rate
Maximum heart rate x training % = target heart rate

For example, if a 50 year old woman wishes to train at 70% of her maximum heart rate, she would use the below calculations:
220 – 50 = 170
170 x 70% = 119

She would thus aim to reach a heart rate of 119 during her exercise in order to work at her target heart rate.

You can also use the Karvonen Formula, which is based on both maximum heart rate and resting heart. Visit *www.sport-fitnessadvisor.com/heart-rate-reserve.html* for more information.

- **Physical Assessment:** The Physical Assessment will provide you with a direct measurement of the improvements you can make in gaining strength as a result of following the exercises in this book. Refer to Chapter 7, page 88 for the Physical Assessment.

- **Waist Size:** To determine your waist-to-height ratio, simply divide your waist size by your height (in inches). A waist-to-height ratio under 50 percent is generally considered healthy.

- **Stamina:** The average person should be able to walk up a flight of stairs or walk once around an outdoor track without becoming out of breath.

  - *12-Minute Walking Test:* Find a measured distance, such as a track, and see how much distance you can cover in 12 minutes. Make sure you challenge yourself, while still being able to carry on intermittent conversation with a partner (see the Talk Test on page 29). Referring to the Rate of Perceived Exertion (RPE) scale on page 29, you should aim to work at around 5–6 during the first two or three times of repeating this test. Thereafter, challenge yourself to reach a 7–8 on the RPE scale. This test is also known as the Cooper Test. You can complete this on a treadmill, too.

  - *Quarter-Mile Timed Test:* Find a measured 400-meter or quarter-mile track. See how long it takes you to cover the specified distance. Aim to work at a 6–7 on the Rate of Perceived Exertion (RPE) scale.

- **Strength:** As you perform the Strength Circuits (see page 94), make note of any improvements you have made. For instance, are you able to perform more reps, or have you continued from beginner to intermediate exercises?

- **Flexibility:** Because levels of flexibility can differ greatly from one individual to the next, it is impossible to provide an average measurement of flexibility. Instead, you should aim to determine what improvements you are making in your Physical Assessment (see page 88) from week to week. This will help you gauge whether you are improving your flexibility based on your body's abilities.

- **Re-Assessment:** Perform the Functional and Physical Assessments again and compare your new results with your original results to determine how much you have improved in your overall strength and function.

CHAPTER SIX

The Exercises

Getting Up From a Chair

Feel it Here Core

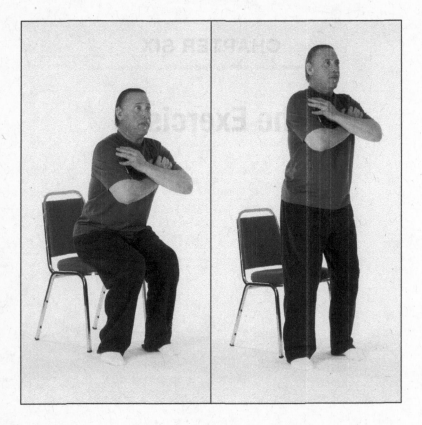

SET-UP

Position yourself on the edge of a chair. Hips should be parallel, or slightly above, knee level. Brace your core and press your feet into the ground.

Standing with Eyes Closed

Feel it Here Full Body

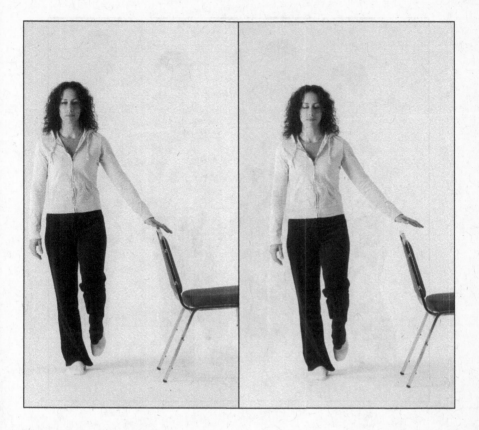

SET-UP

Stand with your feet hip-width apart. You should stand near a wall or partner for safety. For the two-legged test, rest you hands at your side and
close your eyes. With both feet on the ground, feel a natural sway similar
to a tree in the wind. For the one-legged test, close your eyes once your
foot is off the ground. With one foot on the ground, the sway will increase
dramatically with your body wanting to make very quick readjustments to
stabilize.

Heel to Toe Walking

Feel it Here Core, Sides of Legs, Back

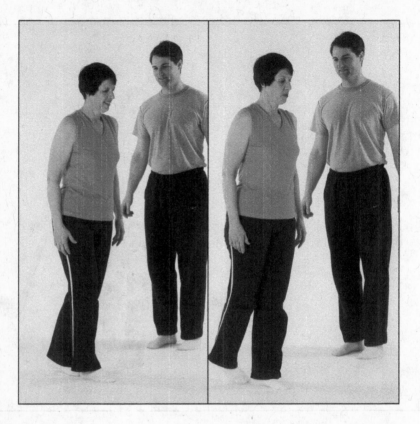

SET-UP

Find a wall or fixed surface prior to beginning this exercise in case you become off balance. Begin with your arms out to the side for added stability. Pick a spot in front of you for focus and begin the movement by placing one foot in front of the other. Experience your upper body attempting to stabilize itself more than when you are in a normal walking position. A dramatic change in stability will occur with one foot in front or behind the other. Take your time and concentrate on the placement of each foot. Repeat backwards toe-to-heel.

Chair Sit

Feel it Here Legs

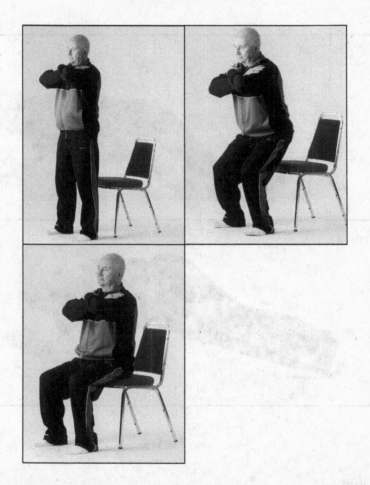

SET-UP

Using the chair as a teaching tool, lower the hips down towards the seat using legs and hips. Hold this position, relax into the chair, repeat. Work on increasing the time held for each rep. A wall can be used if the isometric squat is too much. Position your body against a wall. Walk your hips down the wall by walking your feet out in front of your body. Keep your hips, knees, and toes in line. Maintaining head, shoulder, and tailbone contact with the wall, hold the squatting position as if sitting in a chair. You should not feel pain in your knees. If you do, walk the feet out farther. Breathe into your lower body.

Forward Plank

Feel it Here Stomach, Legs, Shoulders

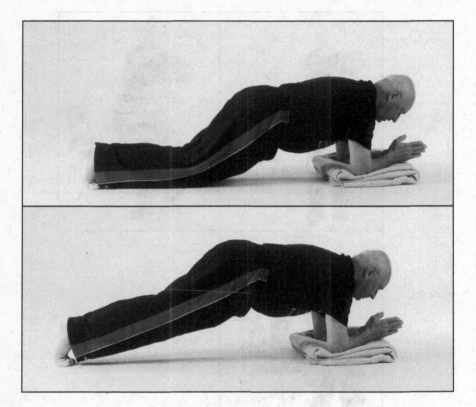

SET-UP

Position your body in the same position as a push-up, but with your hands positioned together in front of your face. To help cue the pulling of the navel to the spine, place a rolled-up towel on your lower back as a bio-feedback tool. Make sure you are breathing through the entire movement. Pull your navel to the lower spine but do not flatten out your lower back. Instead, cue the lower ribs to become "heavy."

Lifting Technique

Feel it Here Legs, Stomach, Spine, Shoulders, Arms.

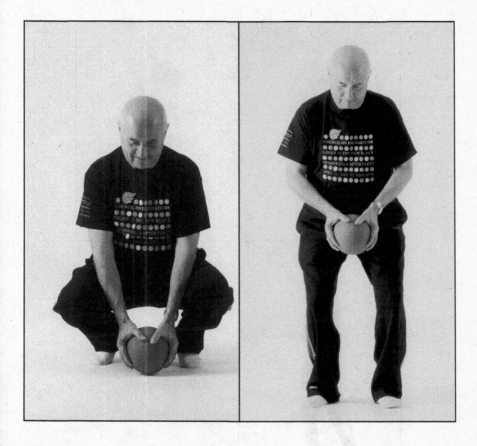

SET-UP

Point your toes to the 11 and 1 o'clock positions. Bend at the hips, knees, and ankles. Keep the object close to your body during the entire motion. Prior to beginning the upward (lifting) movement, brace your stomach and press your feet into the ground, then stand up straight. If you are unable to keep your heels down, it is especially important that you brace your stomach throughout this movement.

Rotating Technique

Feel it Here Hips, Middle Back

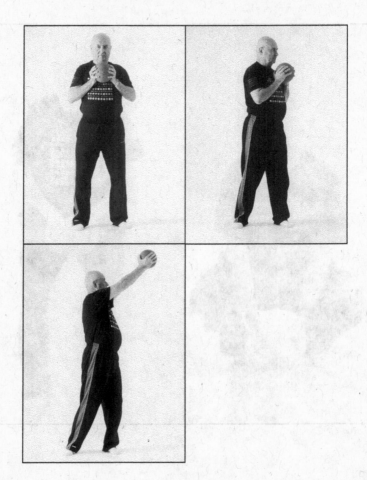

SET-UP

Set up with the same mechanics as for the lifting exercise. Keep the object as close as you can until your hips and spine reach their end points. Be careful not to twist through your lower back.

Squatting Technique

Feel it Here Legs, Back

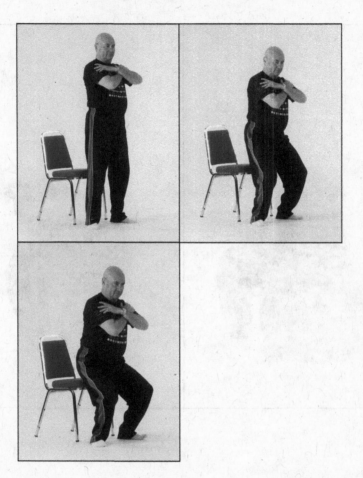

SET-UP

Cross your arms in front of your body. Hands should be resting on the front of your shoulders with elbows relaxed. Brace your stomach. Your toes should be positioned at 11 and 1 o'clock positions to allow proper movement about the hip. Look at a spot on the floor a bit in front of you, but not so much as to be entirely erect. Think about "wrinkling" your groin when squatting. This will force your hips back.

41

Hip Hinging

Feel it Here Lower Spine, Hamstrings

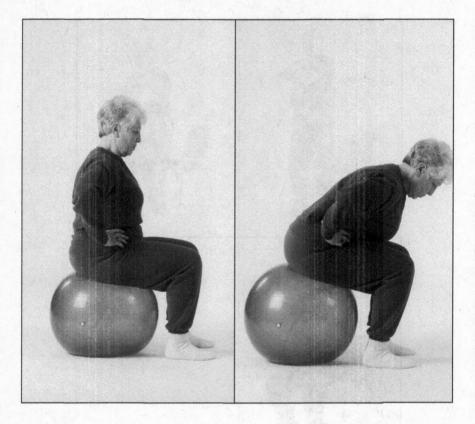

SET-UP

Start the movement from your hips, letting the other parts follow. Feel your upper body positioned over the upper thighs as you "hinge" forward. Brace your stomach, then begin the upward movement, returning to an upright position.

Spinal Whip

Feel it Here Middle Back

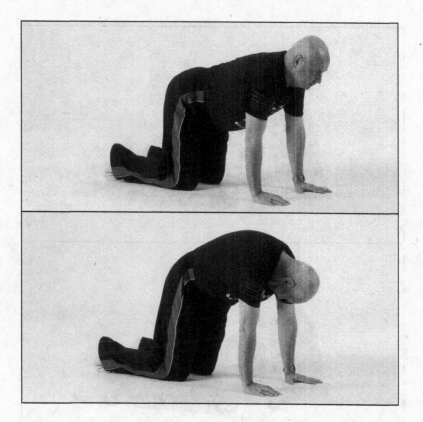

SET-UP

Begin on all fours or standing with your hands on your knees. Rotate from the shoulder blades as they move to the outside of the upper body. Emphasize moving from the middle back through the sternum.

Note: Pay special attention to noticing the difference between your lower, middle, and upper back.

Shoulder Circles

Feel it Here Spine

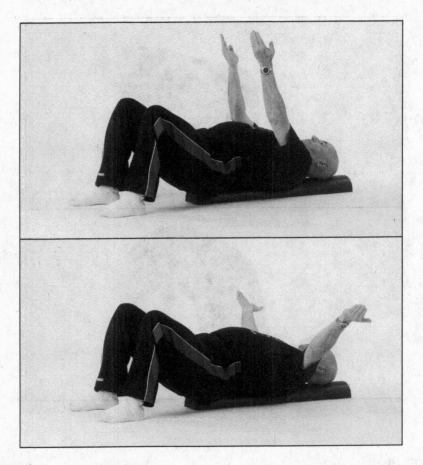

SET-UP

Lay down on the roller with your spine resting in the long position. If you need increased balance during the movement, use a half roller or rolled-up towel. Feel pressure on your spine. Only your head, middle back, and pelvis should be resting in contact with the roller. Initiate smooth circles with your arms as if you have a dinner tray in each hand.

Note: This should be attempted using a half roller first and then using a full roller.

Cranial Release

Feel it Here Neck

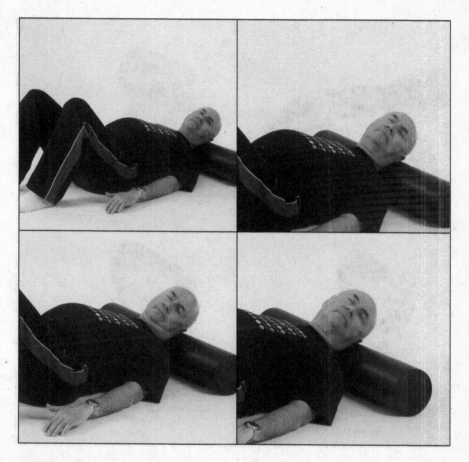

SET-UP

Lay on your back. Position the back of your head, right where it meets the base of your neck, on the roller. You should be in a comfortable position; draw your feet into your hips if needed. Your hands should be relaxed near the sides of your hips. If you need to stabilize the roller, place your hands on the sides of the roller. Rotate your head to the right and left. When rotating your head to the right and left, feel the small space that sits on either side of your head. Keep pressure in the roller by slightly extending your neck, emphasizing proper alignment. *Check out www.meltmethod.com*

Images should be read clockwise.

Sacral Release

Feel it Here Pelvis

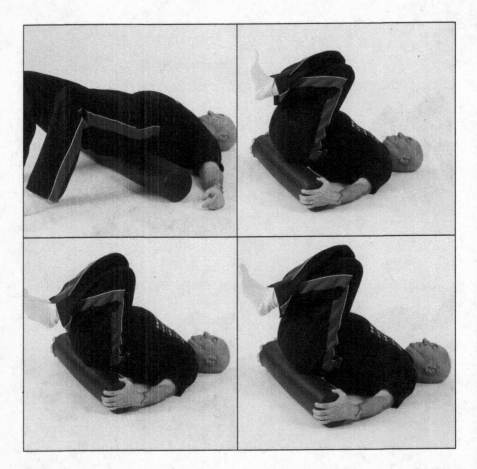

SET-UP

Position your body in a comfortable bridging position on your spine. Elevate your hips and slide the roller on your sacrum. Keeping your ribs heavy, engaging your core, pull one knee at a time up to a position over your hips. Addressing one side of your pelvis at a time, let your knees drift over until you feel a "barrier" or place of irritability. Once found, gently make circles with your knees both ways, then switch to the other side. *Check out www.meltmethod.com*

Images should be read clockwise.

MELT Ball Series

Feel it Here Small Joints

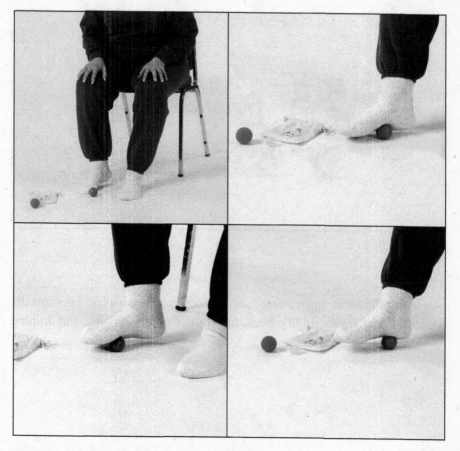

SET-UP

Apply balls to joint and soft surfaces allowing the joints/tissues to decompress and open. Compression is one of our body's enemies as we age. Similar patterns of position point pressing can be applied to the hands and feet. Do not let the balls sink into the soft tissue spaces between the joints—nerves sit there. Check out *www.meltmethod.com*

Images should be read clockwise.

Sleeping with Pillows

Feel it Here Back

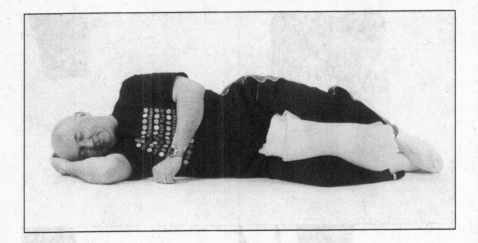

SET-UP
Position pillows in spaces that "unload" joints and muscles: between the knees, under the ribs/middle back, under the front of the hips, and draping the arms.

Ankle Pumps

Feel it Here Front of Shins, Calves

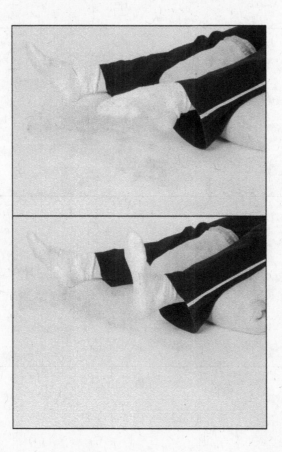

SET-UP

Gently point and flex the foot, reaching out through the front of the big toe.
Pull the toes back by pushing through the heel.

49

Foam Roller Scissor Stretch

Feel it Here Core, Lower Back

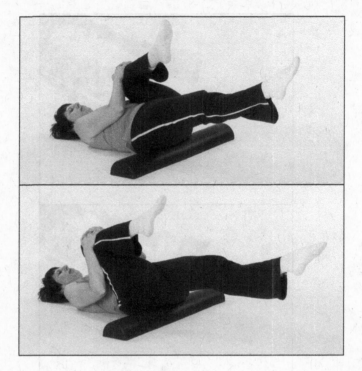

SET-UP

Lay on your back with your knees bent and feet close to your hips. Press your feet into the floor, then elevate your hips. Slide a foam roller (or very thick towel) beneath your tailbone/sacrum. Keeping your ribs heavy, pull one knee to your chest and hold. Extend the leg next, keeping ribs heavy and engaging the core. The sacrum is the flattish bone that positions itself directly below the lower back. Place the palm of your hand on the sacrum; it should fit nicely. The roller sits between the lower back and sacrum. *Check out www.meltmethod.com*

Roll and Hold

Feel it Here Upper and Lower Spine

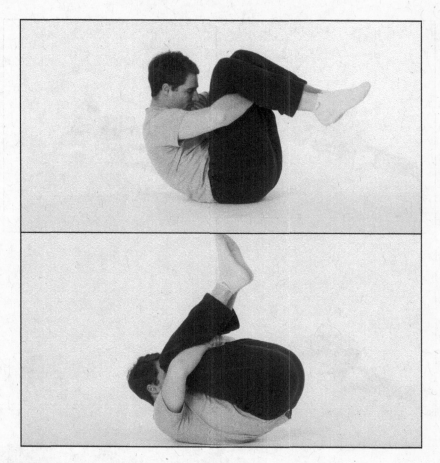

SET-UP
Tuck the knees into your chest and rock back and forth.

Ribcage Opener

Feel it Here Groin, Back, Shoulders

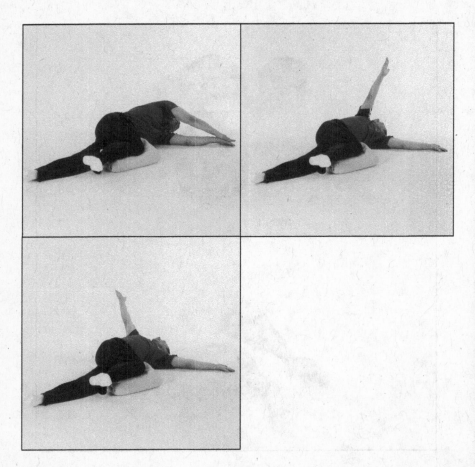

SET-UP

Lay on the ground and position a rolled-up towel or foam roller under your knee. Start with your hands together. Press your knees into the object, then initiate rotation with your hand. Follow the rotation down the arm until you feel it through your ribcage.

Thoracic Flex on Roller

Feel it Here Middle Spine, Abdominals

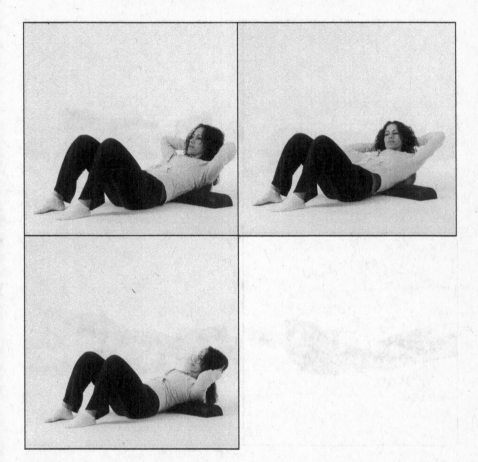

SET-UP

You can use a full roller, half roller, or thick, rolled-up towel. Position the roller immediately below your shoulder blades. Your elbows should be pointed to the sides. Feel the foam roller pressing against your middle spine. Keep your ribs heavy into the ground so the core muscles are active and working through the entire motion. Your front abs will be working the entire time but the latter muscles, namely the obliques, are the actual movers.

Note: This should be attempted using a half roller first and then using a full roller.

53

Prone Extension Lifts

Feel it Here Middle and Lower Back, Hips

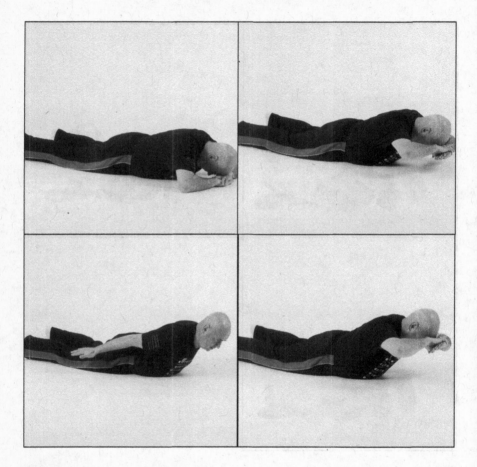

SET-UP

Gently press the front of your lower body into the ground. Initiate the lifting movement from your head, then shoulders, middle back, and lower back. Hold, then release slowly.

Images should be read clockwise.

Heel to Toe Rocks

Feel it Here Full Body

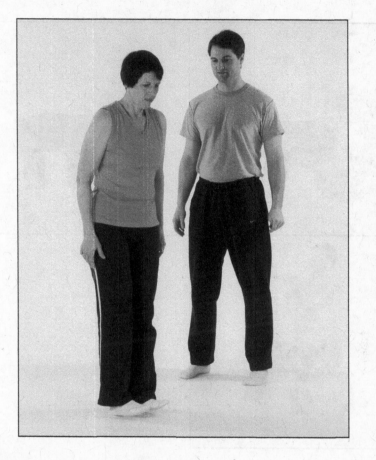

SET-UP

Partner rocks back and forth from the toes to heels as you provide support if needed.

Physio-Ball Walk-Up

Feel it Here Legs, Hips, Core

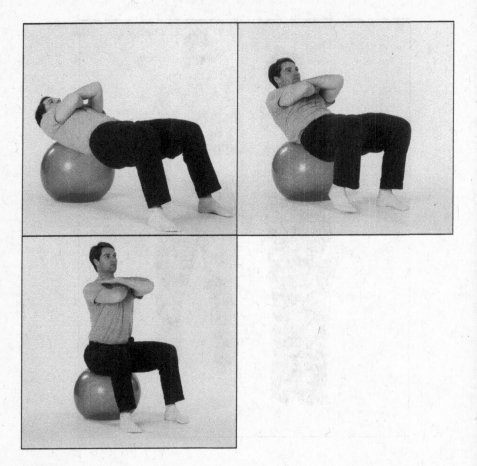

SET-UP

Position your hips on top of the physio-ball. Brace your core. Walk up the ball using your full foot. Keeping the feet wider adds stability if you feel off balance during the up or down phases.

Clock Series: Single Foot Touches

Feel it Here Legs, Hips

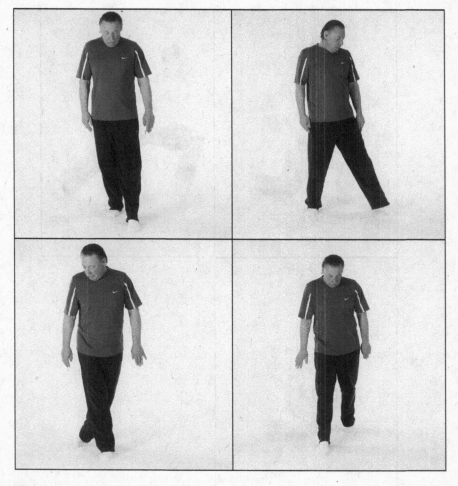

SET-UP

Imagine you are standing in the center of a clock face. Touch 2–3 numbers around the clock. As you become more comfortable, touch more numbers, then switch feet.

Images should be read clockwise.

Clock Lunge

Feel it Here Hips, Legs

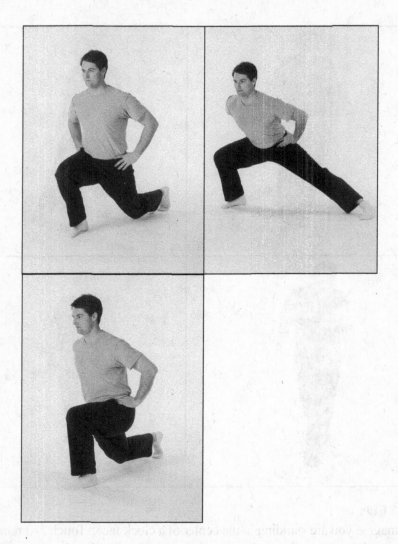

SET-UP

Imagine you are standing in the middle of a clock face. Lunge to various positions on the clock face. Lunging needs to be executed with proper movement at the hip and knee. Sit the hips down and back into each number on the clock face.

Physio-Ball Foot Lifts

Feel it Here Hips, Legs

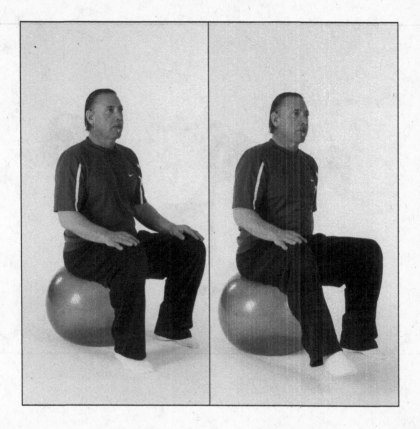

SET-UP

Sit on the very top of the physio-ball. You should feel as if you are sitting slightly higher than on a regular chair and a bit more open in the front of the hips. Use the hip hinging cue (see page 42) to find the back alignment necessary to maintain positioning and stability. Feel braced through the core. This will stabilize your back and hips before you lift your foot. Lift one foot off the floor, hold. Work on shifting your body weight slowly to one foot prior to lifting the opposing knee/foot. Use a mirror or partner to accomplish.

Doggy Door

Feel it Here Groin, Hips

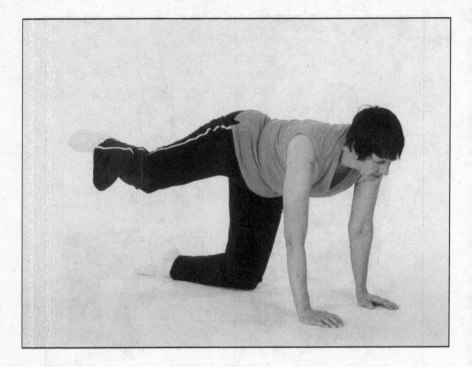

SET-UP

Keep you core active to stabilize your back and hips. Keeping the non-lifting hip firm into the ground, lift the opposite knee with the outside hip muscle. Be careful not to shift your weight to the non-working side.

Inch Worm Walk-Up

Feel it Here Shoulders, Core, Legs

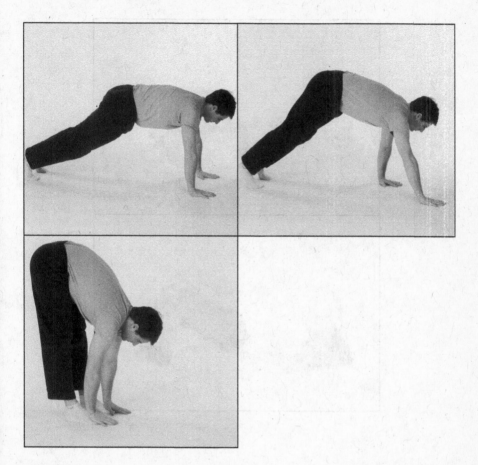

SET-UP

Beginning in a pike position, walk your hands forward until you reach the starting position for a push-up. Brace your stomach, then walk your hands back toward the feet. Do not allow your back to sag once the push-up position is reached. Keeping your hands moving together during this movement is important.

Double Leg Bridge

Feel it Here Back of Legs, Hips, Back

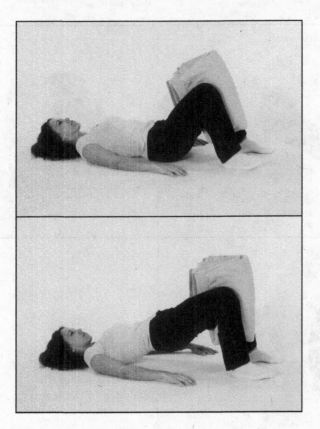

SET-UP

Starting on your back, press the feet into the ground to feel the leg muscles contract. Brace your core, then lift the hips to form an alignment between the knees, hips, and shoulders.

Pelvic Tilt

Feel it Here Obliques, Abdominals, Lower Back

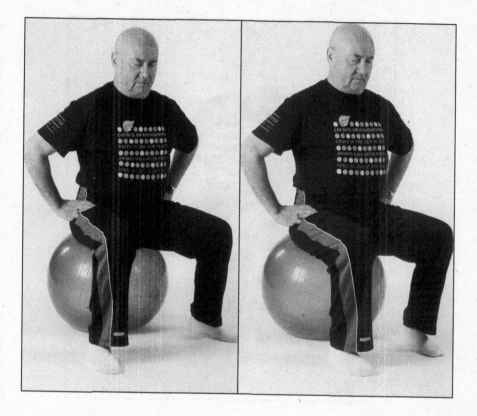

SET-UP
Sit on a physio-ball with both knees bent and your feet flat on the floor. Tilt your pelvis in line with your hips. You may also place your hand on your belly and lower back to facilitate movement. Feel the difference between this exercise and the kegel exercise on page 64. You should notice a distinct anatomical difference between the lower back and ribs.

Kegel

Feel it Here Pelvic Floor, Core

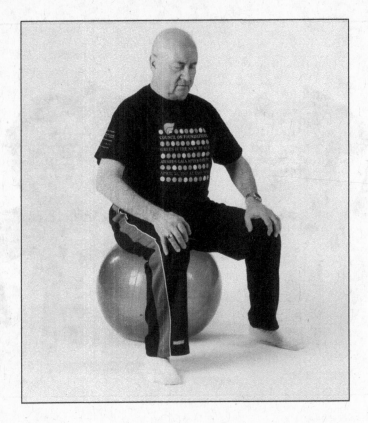

SET-UP

While keeping the lower back quiet and relaxed, squeeze your pelvic floor muscles in and up towards the pelvis. Imagine there is a balloon attached to your pelvic floor and it is rising. Try this exercise on the floor first to take surrounding muscles out of the learning curve.

Bent Knee Hamstring

Feel it Here Back of Upper/Middle Leg

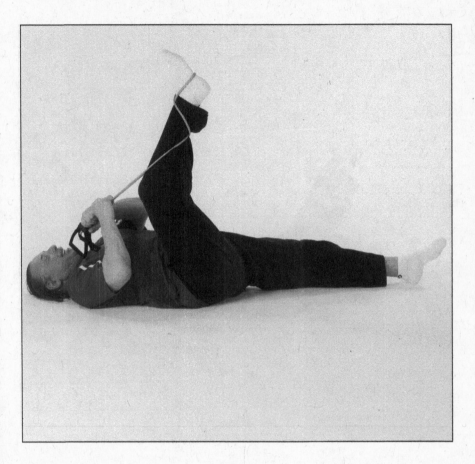

SET-UP

Lay on your back and draw one knee into your chest. Wrap the towel or stretch cord around the arch of your foot. Pull your ankle toward the back of your hip without letting your hip move. Hold the pressure for five seconds. Release and breathe out slowly. Repeat the movement from the newly obtained position.

65

Adductors with Band

Feel it Here Inner Groin, Hip

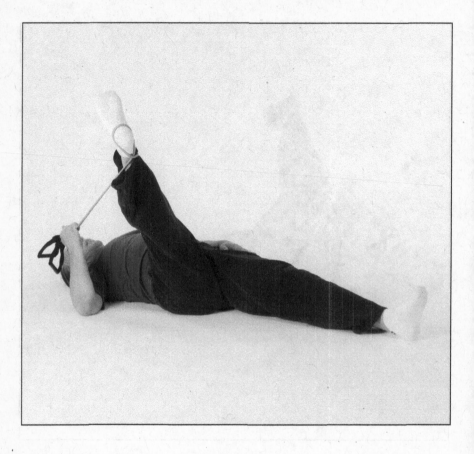

SET-UP

Wrap the towel or stretch cord around the ankle of the leg you want to stretch. Keeping the non-stretching leg down on the floor, press your ankle in toward your body against resistance, and release. Hold the pressure for five seconds. Release and breathe out slowly. Repeat the movement from the newly obtained position.

Abductors

Feel it Here Outer Hip, Obliques, Lower Back

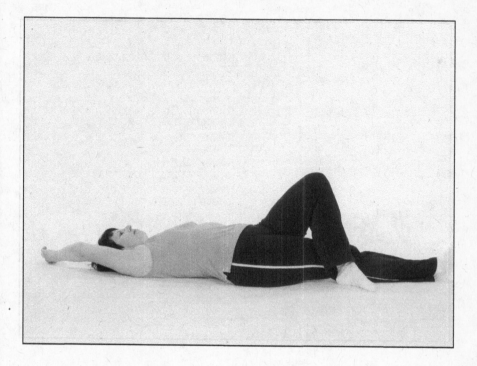

SET-UP

Keeping the non-stretching leg down on the floor, cross the opposite ankle over the leg, pressing against the knee. Hold the pressure for five seconds. Release and breathe out slowly. Repeat the movement from the newly obtained position.

Quads/Hip Flexors

Feel it Here Front of Leg

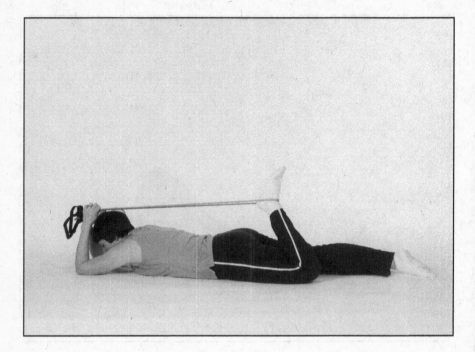

SET-UP

This exercise can be done lying on your stomach or on your side. Lying on your stomach decreases the likelihood that you will arch your lower back during the stretch. Hold the pressure for 5 seconds, then release and breathe out slowly. Repeat the movement from the newly obtained position. If you are feeling the stretch in your lower back, place a pillow or rolled-up towel under the front of your hips for support. If you are feeling the stretch in the front of your knee, place the towel under the front of your knee and continue with the stretch.

Posterior Neck Stretch

Feel it Here Back of Neck

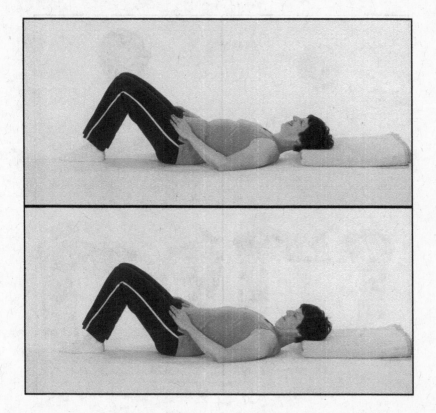

SET-UP

This exercise can be executed lying on your back or standing against a wall. If lying on your back, roll up a towel and place it above the point where your head meets your neck. For the standing version, the towel should be slightly larger to stabilize your neck. Roll the towel and place it in the same position previously mentioned. Both stretches require a gentle tucking of the chin in the front of the neck while "lengthening" the back of the head up and over the chin.

Lateral Neck Stretch

Feel it Here Neck, Shoulder

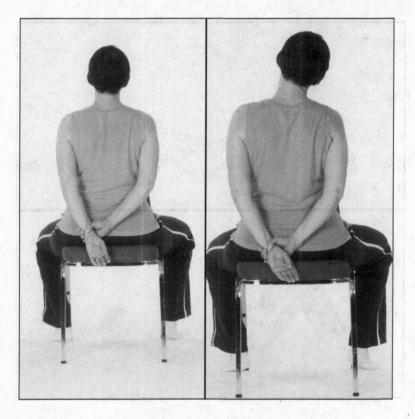

SET-UP

Sit with the arm of the shoulder to be stretched placed behind you. Gently drop your ear to your other shoulder. Then, grab the wrist of the shoulder/ neck area being stretched and hold. Relax the opposite shoulder by breathing deeply into the side being stretched. Allow your head to return to neutral before releasing the wrist.

Knee to Forehead

Feel it Here Hips

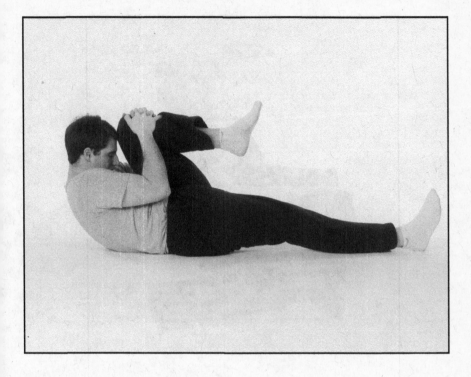

SET-UP

Tighten up the stomach. Draw the knee towards the chest, grabbing the knee with two hands.

Glutes

Feel it Here Outer Hip, Lower Back, Hamstrings

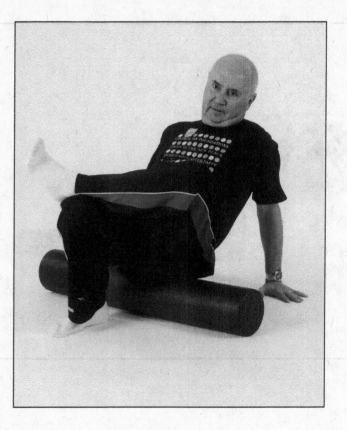

SET-UP

Position your outer hip on the roller. Apply pressure into the roller with the hip, and slowly rotate the hip from the knee.

Straight Leg Stretch

Feel it Here Back of Leg

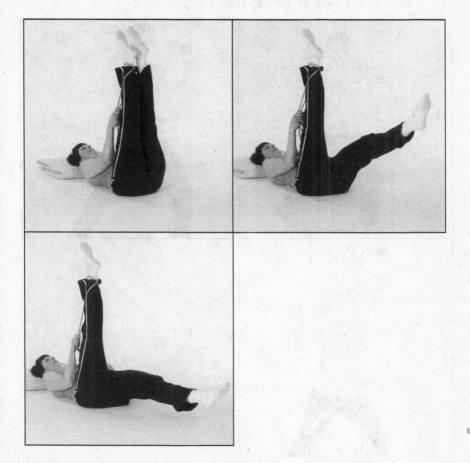

SET-UP

This stretch can be done using a door frame or stretch cord (as shown). Both variations are great stretches for the back of the leg.

73

Lateral Lunge with Shoulder Press

Feel it Here Hips, Knees, Ankles

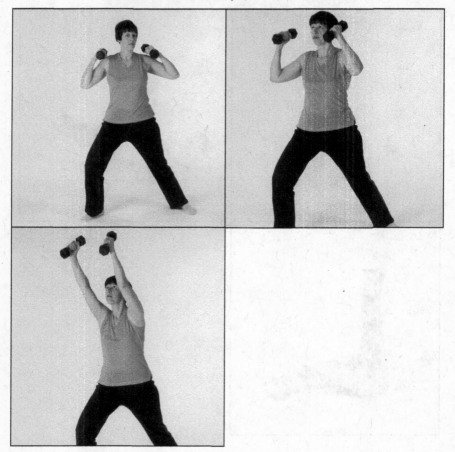

SET-UP

Lunge to the side, sitting back into the exercise. Upon returning to the starting position, press the dumbbells across the body. Be sure to keep your back straight and your shoulders squared forward.

Band Rows

Feel it Here Middle Back, Arms

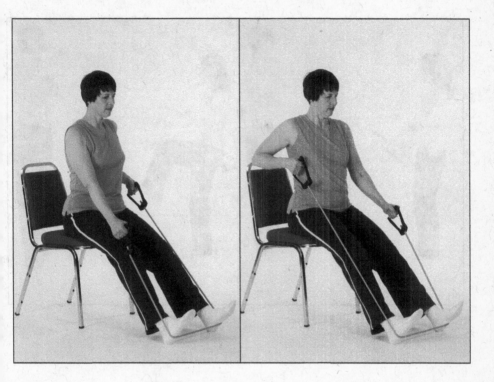

SET-UP

Execute the movement by drawing one elbow back while "punching" the opposite arm forward. The objective is to learn rotation and build strength in the traditionally weak core and shoulder girdle. This is important for posture during walking and sitting. If you feel discomfort in your neck, concentrate on relaxing the shoulder blades back and down.

Band Pulls with One Knee Up

Feel it Here Core, Arms, Chest, Legs

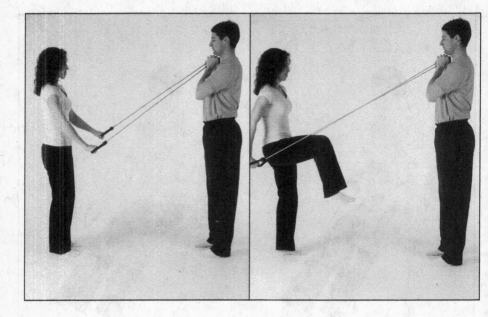

SET-UP

In a standing position, pull your knee upward towards your chest while pulling the arms to the sides of your body. Keep your ribs heavy and core contracted during each pressing repetition. Breathe out during each pressing rep and breathe in upon returning to the starting position.

Alphabet Series: W's

Feel it Here Middle Back

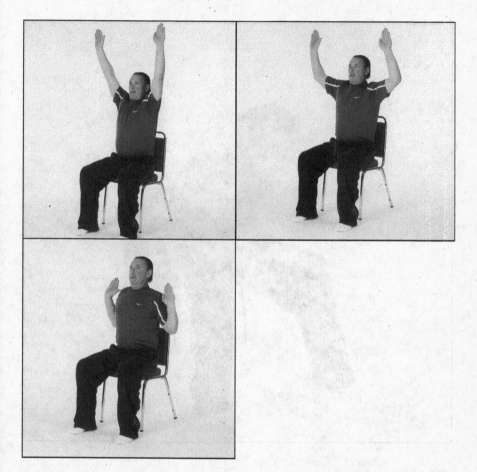

SET-UP

Sit upright on a sturdy surface. Squeeze your shoulder blades back and down. Draw both elbows down and back into the middle spine. Hold, then release.

Alphabet Series: Y's

Feel it Here Middle and Lower Back

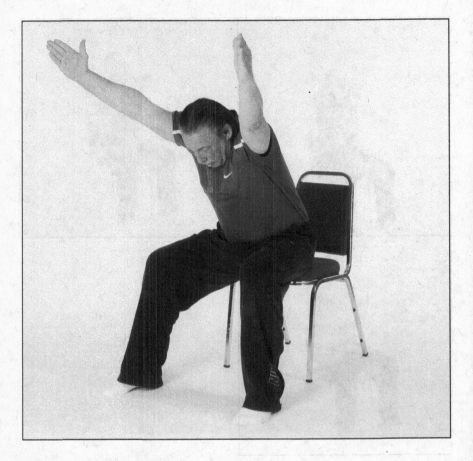

SET-UP

Sit upright on a sturdy surface. Squeeze your shoulder blades back and down. Draw both arms up and straight out in front of your body at a 45 degree angle.

Alphabet Series: T's

Feel it Here Middle Back, Behind Shoulders

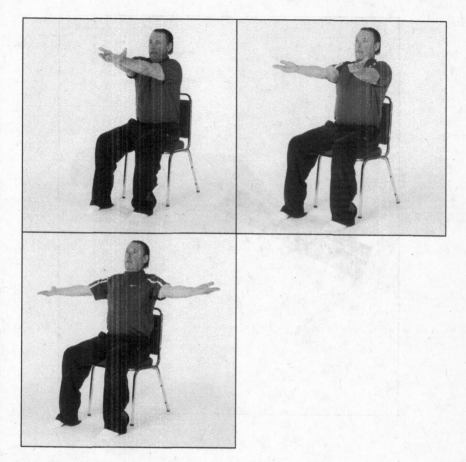

SET-UP

Sit upright on a sturdy surface. Squeeze your shoulder blades back and down. Draw both arms out from the mid-line of the body with palms up.

79

Stability Hold in Push-Up

Feel it Here Core, Shoulders, Legs

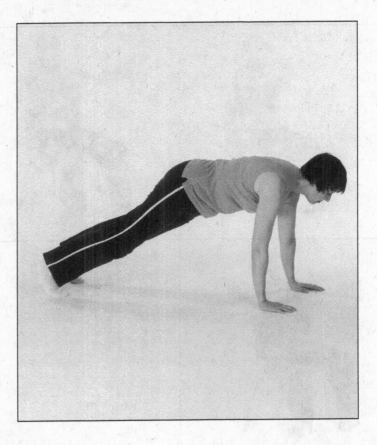

SET-UP

Assume a push-up position. Brace your core, be strong through your spine, and balanced on your hands and feet.

Standard Lunge with Bicep Curl

Feel it Here Stomach, Obliques

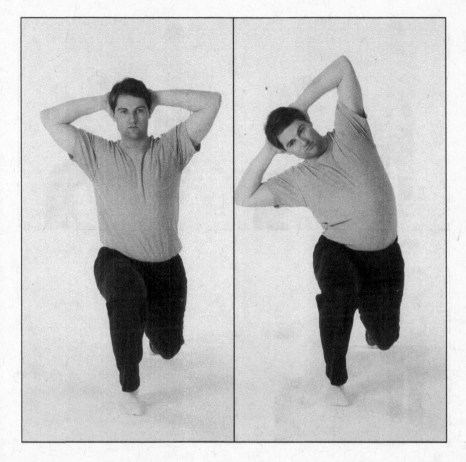

SET-UP

Lunging is nothing more than an exaggerated step. For an advanced lunge (shown, right), make sure your hips are stable and then flex your trunk to the same side as the front leg. Begin to initiate the bicep curl once your lunging motion is completed.

Band Presses with Two Arms

Feel it Here Chest, Shoulders, Arms

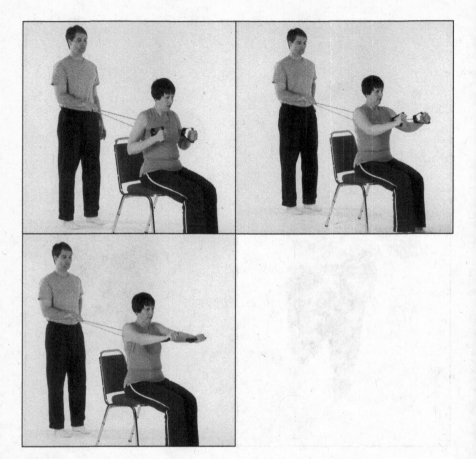

SET-UP

Position your body in a standing position in a normal stance or a split stance. Press your hands out in front until your elbows are fully extended. Keep the ribs heavy and core contracted during each pressing repetition. Breathe out during each extension and breathe in upon return to the starting position. This exercise can also be done while sitting (shown above) in an upright position on either a ball or a bench.

Chopping Movements

Feel it Here Core, Hips

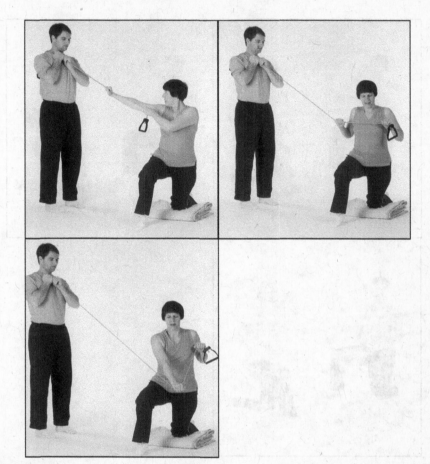

SET-UP

Chop across your body over a trailing, kneeling leg. Your front knee is on the ground on a towel or other comfortable item. Pull the band into your body, then push it down and out with the trail hand. Keep your spine neutral by concentrating on bracing your stomach and stabilizing the hips. Think about moving around a stable pillar in your spine.

Exercise provided by St. John's, AAHFRP, FMS

Lifting Movements

Feel it Here Core, Hips

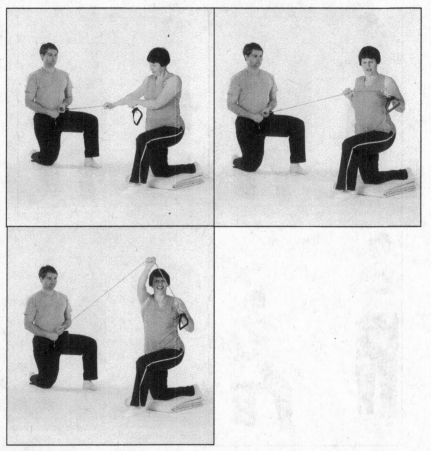

SET-UP

You will be lifting across your body over a trailing knee on the ground. The front knee should be aligned with your hip. Pull the band into your body, then push it up and out with the trailing hand. Keep your spine neutral by concentrating on bracing your stomach and stabilizing the hips. Think about moving around a stable pillar in your spine.

Exercise provided by St. John's, AAHFRP, FMS

CHAPTER SEVEN

Exercise Programs and Progressions

Programs

Introductory
AM
- Start the Self-Treatment and Massage progression (see page 90)
- Start the Posture Basics progression (see page 90)

PM
- Weekly: Complete the initial Functional Assessment (see page 88)
- Complete the initial Physical Fitness Assessment (see page 88)

Beginner Fibromyalgia Program
AM
- Start the Beginner: Mobility progression (see page 91)
- Start the Upper or Lower Flexibility progression (see page 93)

PM
- Start the Balance progression (see page 92)

Intermediate Fibromyalgia Program

AM

- Start the Intermediate: Mobility progression (see page 91) or the Stability progression (see page 92)
- Practice Upper Flexibility progression (see page 93)
- Practice the Balance progression (see page 92)

PM

- Practice Balance progression (see page 92)
- Practice your favorite Mobility progression (see pages 91)

Advanced Fibromyalgia Program

AM

- Start the Strength Circuit (see page 94)
- Re-test the Physical Fitness Assessment (page 88)
- Start the Strength progression (see page 94)

PM

- Practice the Balance progression (see page 92)

Supplemental Program

- Start the Techniques progression (see page 89)

Progressions

Rep (or repetition) refers to the number of times you perform a movement.

Sets represent how many times you complete a given number of repetitions of a group of exercises (also known as Progressions).

RPE refers to Rate of perceived Exertion. See page 29 for details.

Assessments

INITIAL EVALUATION DATE (WEEK 1): _____

MID-POINT EVALUATION DATE (WEEK 4): _____

SUMMARY EVALUATION DATE (WEEK 9): _____

FUNCTIONAL ASSESSMENT	COMPLETE? (Yes/No)	DISCOMFORT? (Yes/No)	NOTE DIFFICULTY
Getting Up From a Chair			
Standing with Eyes Closed			
Heel to Toe Walking			

PHYSICAL FITNESS ASSESSMENT	GOAL	INITIAL	MID-POINT	SUMMARY
Chair Sit	Achieve movement without using handles			
Forward Plank	Achieve neutral spine without allowing the back to sag			
Lifting Technique	Keep the back straight without pain			
Rotating Technique	Complete rotation without discomfort			
Squatting Technique	Bend hips, knees, and ankles together			

Techniques

Reps: 10
Sets: 2
RPE: 5/10

Exercise	Page #	Equipment
Lifting Technique	39	weighted object
Rotating Technique	40	weighted object
Squatting Technique	41	chair

Posture Basics

Reps: 15
Sets: 1
RPE: 3/10

Exercise	Page #	Equipment
Hip Hinging	42	physio-ball
Spinal Whip	43	
Shoulder Circles	44	foam roller or rolled towel

Self-Treatment and Massage

Reps: 15
Sets: 1
RPE: 2/10

Exercise	Page #	Equipment
Cranial Release	45	foam roller or rolled towel
Sacral Release	46	foam roller or rolled towel
MELT Ball Series	47	foam roller or rolled towel
Sleeping with Pillows	48	foam roller or rolled towel

Mobility

Beginner Segment
Reps: 12
Sets: 1-2
RPE: 4/10

Exercise	Page #	Equipment
Ankle Pumps	49	rolled towel
Foam Roller Scissor Stretch	50	foam roller or rolled towel
Ribcage Opener	52	foam roller or rolled towel
Thoracic Flex on Roller	53	foam roller or rolled towel

Intermediate Segment
Reps: 12
Sets: 2
RPE: 5/10

Exercise	Page #	Equipment
Foam Roller Scissor Stretch	50	foam roller or rolled towel
Ribcage Opener	52	foam roller or rolled towel
Thoracic Flex on Roller	53	foam roller or rolled towel
Prone Extension Lifts	54	
Roll and Hold	51	

Balance

Reps/Seconds: 10
Sets: 2
RPE: 5/10

Exercise	Page #	Equipment
Clock Series: Single Foot Touches	57	
Physio-Ball Foot Lifts	59	physio-ball
Heel to Toe Rocks	55	
Physio-Ball Walk-Up	56	physio-ball
Clock Lunge	58	
Doggy Door	60	

Stability

Reps/Seconds: 8-10
Sets: 2
RPE: 6/10

Exercise	Page #	Equipment
Double Leg Bridge	62	rolled towel
Pelvic Tilt	63	physio-ball
Kegel	64	physio-ball
Inch Worm Walk-Up	61	

Flexibility: Lower Body

Reps/Seconds: 15-25
Sets: 2
RPE: 7/10

Exercise	Page #	Equipment
Bent Knee Hamstring	65	theraband
Adductors with Band	66	theraband
Abductors	67	
Quads/Hip Flexors	68	theraband
Glutes	72	foam roller
Straight Leg Stretch	73	theraband

Flexibility: Upper Body

Reps/Seconds: 10
Sets: 2
RPE: 3/10

Exercise	Page #	Equipment
Knee to Forehead	71	
Posterior Neck Stretch	69	rolled towel
Lateral Neck Stretch	70	chair

Strength

Note: Be sure to complete these exercises through a pain-free range of motion as they become progressively more difficult from the beginning to the end of this progression.

Reps: 12
Sets: 2
RPE: 6/10

Exercise	Page #	Equipment
Band Rows	75	theraband
Alphabet Series	77-79	chair
Lifting Movements	84	theraband, towel
Chopping Movements	83	theraband, towel
Stability Hold in Push-Up	80	
Band Presses with Two Arms	82	theraband, towel
Band Pulls with One Knee Up	76	theraband
Lateral Lunge with Shoulder Press or Standard Lunge with Bicep Curl	74, 81	dumbbells

RESOURCES

Arthritis Foundation
arthritis.org

Centers for Disease Control and Prevention (CDC)
www.cdc.gov

Fibromyalgia.com
www.fibromyalgia.com

Fibromyalgia Network
www.fmnetnews.com

Fibromyalgia Symptoms
www.fibromyalgia-symptoms.org

Fibromyalgia Treatment
www.fibromyalgia-treatment.com

The MELT Method
www.meltmethod.com

National Fibromyalgia Association (NFA)
www.fmaware.org

The National Institute of Arthritis and Musculoskeletal and Skin Diseases (NIAMS)
www.niams.nih.gov

U.S. National Library of Medicine
www.ncbi.nlm.nih.gov/pubmedhealth

ABOUT THE AUTHORS

William Smith, MS, NSCA, CSCS, MEPD, completed his B.S. in exercise science at Western Michigan University followed by a master's degree in education and a post-graduate program at Rutgers University. In 1993, Will began coaching triathletes and working with athletes and post-rehab clientele. He was a Division I Collegiate Strength Coach and has been competing in triathlons and marathons since 1998, recently finishing the Steelhead Half Ironman in Michigan in 5 hours and 22 minutes. Will founded Will Power and Fitness Associates and currently consults for fitness, healthcare, and wellness centers in New York and New Jersey. The Director of the Professional Development Institute, Will has also co-authored a book on triathlon training (*Tri-Power*, 2007).

Jo Brielyn is a freelance writer and author. She is a contributing writer for Hatherleigh Press and has published works in several print and online publications. Jo also owns and maintains the Creative Kids Ideas (www.creativekidsideas.com) and Good for Your Health (www.good-for-yourhealth.com) websites. For more information about Jo's upcoming projects or to contact her, visit www.JoBrielyn.com. Jo resides in Central Florida with her husband and two daughters.

Zinovy Meyler, DO, is the Co-Director of the Interventional Spine Program and an attending physician at Princeton Spine and Joint Center in Princeton, NJ. Dr. Meyler is a board certified, fellowship-trained physician specializing in the non-operative treatment of spine, joint, and muscle pain with emphasis on image-guided interventional spine and joint procedures.